Keto Diet

The Keto Way Cookbook

Books By Francine Brown

Keto Diet: Keto Diet Steps to The Keto Way For Rapid Weight Loss And Good Health

Keto Diet: Keto Diet Steps To The Keto Way For People On The Go

Keto Diet: The Keto Way For Singles

Keto Diet: The Keto Way Cookbook For the Holidays

Weight Loss And Diet: Weight Loss And Keeping it Off Successfully

Grief: My Only Child Died! Grief And How To Live Your Everyday Life

Free Delicious Easy Keto Recipe Ebook

https://francinebrownbooks.com

Keto Diet

The Keto Way Cookbook for Singles

Author
Francine Brown

Table of Contents

Introduction
Chapter 1: Breakfast

Keto Avocado Toast
Chocolate Chip Waffles
Egg Crepes with Avocados
Breakfast Blueberry Coconut Smoothie
Vegan Chocolate Smoothie
Power Green Smoothie
Kiwi Coconut Smoothie
Mixed Nuts & Smoothie Breakfast
Superfood Red Smoothie
Coconut Shake with Avocado
Breakfast Cheesy Sausage
Ham and Cheese Pockets
Clementine and Pistachio Ricotta
Gingerbread-Spiced Breakfast Smoothie
Vegan Breakfast Muffins
Vegan Breakfast Biscuits
Vegan Breakfast Sausages
Quick Breakfast Yogurt

Chapter 2: Lunch

Cheesy Spinach
Creamy Brussels Sprout
Broccoli Stir Fry
Beef Roast
Almond Cinnamon Beef Meatballs
Creamy Beef Stroganoff
Baked Chicken Fajitas
Baked Chicken Wings
Chicken with Spinach Broccoli
Delicious Bacon Chicken
Mexican Chicken
Beef Casserole

Kelp noodle salad
Spicy Satay Tofu Salad
Mexican Beef with Zucchini
Mexican Beef
7 minute noodles
Cheese head gnocchi
Fettuccine
Roasted Onions and Green Beans
Green Bean Roast
Buttery Lamb Chops
Lemon Herb Lamb Chops
Fennel Grill Pork Chops

Chapter 3: Dinner

Cauliflower Rice
Spinach & Cauliflower Soup
Oriental red cabbage salad
Broccoli salad with fresh dill
Stuffed Zucchini
Coconut pasta
Spinach pasta
Avocado Fries
Mushroom Zoodle Pasta
Quick Veggie Protein Bowl
Tasty Green Salad
Asparagus and Artichoke Salad
Soy flour noodles
Shrimp Scampi
Grilled Salmon
Shrimp and Garlic
Salmon Patties
Beef Stew

Chapter 4: Snacks

Coconut Cheesecake
Raspberry Nut Truffles

Chocolate Cakes
Blueberry Ice Pops
Strawberry Vanilla Shake
Vanilla Ice Cream
Chia and Blackberry Pudding
Almond Butter Fat Bombs
Mixed Berry Trifle
Walnut Cookies
Cinnamon and Turmeric Latte
Chocolate Bark with Almonds
Vanilla Berry Mug Cake
Pumpkin Spice Mug Cake
Berry Acai Smoothie
Choco-Coco Milk Shake
Nutty Choco Milk Shake
Choco Milk Smoothie
Creamy Choco Shake
Baby Kale and Yogurt Smoothie
Raspberry Chocolate Fudge

Conclusion

Introduction

As a single person do you want to start the ketogenic diet lifestyle but not sure where to start? Are you struggling to find delicious recipes just for one, Keep reading!

This Singles Cookbook contains amazingly delicious keto recipes for one that get you going in a jiffy for your single keto lifestyle.

These mouth-watering recipes are ideal for any occasion, and they are great for your health. Ditching carbs do not mean ditching yummy treats, and with these recipes, you will see that for yourself.

The ketogenic diet has been successfully practiced for almost a century, and it has proven to be the ultimate long-term diet for any person. The keto diet is super adaptable, and the tasty meals are pretty endless.

Enjoy reading!

CHAPTER 1: BREAKFAST

Keto Avocado Toast

Prep time: 5 minutes/ Cook time: 2 minutes / Serves 1

Ingredients
- 1 tablespoon sunflower oil
- ½ cup parmesan cheese, shredded
- 1 medium avocado, sliced
- Sea salt, to taste
- 2 slices cauliflower bread

Directions:
1. Heat oil in a pan and cook cauliflower bread slices for about 2 minutes per side.
2. Season avocado with sea salt and place on the cauliflower bread.
3. Top with parmesan cheese and microwave for about 2 minutes.

Nutritional information:
Calories 141, Carbs 4.5 g, Fats 10 g, Protein 10.6 g

Chocolate Chip Waffles

Prep time: 30 minutes/ Cook time: 0 minutes / Serves 2

Ingredients:
- 3 scoop vanilla protein powder
- 3 pinch pink Himalayan sea salt
- 150 grams sugar-free chocolate chips
- 3 large eggs, separated
- 3 tablespoons butter, melted

Directions:
1. Mix together egg yolks, vanilla protein powder and butter in a bowl.
2. Whisk together egg whites thoroughly in another bowl and transfer to the egg yolks mixture.
3. Add the sugar-free chocolate chips and a pinch of pink salt.
4. Transfer this mixture to the waffle maker and cook according to manufacturer's instructions.

Nutritional information:
Calories 301, Carbs 6.9 g, Fats 18.8 g, Protein 29.9 g

Egg Crepes with Avocados

Prep time: 15 minutes/ Cook time: 3 minutes / Serves 2

Ingredients:
- 4 eggs
- 2 large avocados, thinly sliced
- 3 teaspoon olive oil
- 1 ½ cup alfalfa sprouts
- 4 slices turkey breast cold cuts, shredded

Directions:
1. Heat olive oil over medium heat in a pan and crack in the eggs.
2. Spread the eggs lightly with the spatula and cook for about 3 minutes on both sides.
3. Dish out the egg crepe and top with turkey breast, alfalfa sprouts and avocado.
4. Roll up tightly and serve warm.

Nutritional information:
Calories 372, Carbs 9.3 g, Fats 25.9 g, Protein 27.2 g

Breakfast Blueberry Coconut Smoothie

Prep time: 5 minutes/ Cook time: 0 minutes / Serves 1
Ingredients:
- 1 avocado, pitted and sliced
- 2 cups blueberries
- 1 cup coconut milk
- 6 tbsp coconut cream
- 2 tsp erythritol
- 2 tbsp coconut flakes

Directions:
1. Combine the avocado slices, blueberries, coconut milk, coconut cream, erythritol, and ice cubes in a smoothie maker and blend until smooth.
2. Pour the smoothie into drinking glasses, and serve sprinkled with coconut flakes.

Nutritional information:
Calories 492, Fat 36.3g, Carbs 8.6g, Protein 9.6g

Vegan Chocolate Smoothie

Prep time: 10 minutes/ Cook time: 0 minutes / Serves 1

Ingredients
- ¼ cup pumpkin seeds
- ¾ cup coconut milk
- ¼ cup water
- 1 ½ cups watercress
- 2 tsp vegan protein powder
- 1 tbsp chia seeds
- 1 tbsp unsweetened cocoa powder

Directions
1. In a blender, add all ingredients except for the chia seeds and process until creamy and uniform. Place into two glasses, dust with chia seeds and chill before serving.

Nutritional information:
Calories 335, Fats 29.7g, Carbs: 5.7g, Protein: 6.5g

Power Green Smoothie

Prep time: 5 minutes/ Cook time: 0 minutes / Serves 1

Ingredients
- 1 cup collard greens, chopped
- 3 stalks celery, chopped
- 1 ripe avocado, skinned, pitted, sliced
- 1 cup ice cubes
- 2 cups spinach, chopped
- 1 large cucumber, peeled and chopped
- Chia seeds to garnish

Directions
2. Add the collard greens, celery, avocado, and ice cubes in a blender, and blend for 50 seconds. Add the spinach and cucumber, and process for another 40 seconds until smooth.
3. Transfer the smoothie into glasses, garnish with chia seeds and serve right away.

Nutritional information:
Calories 187, Fat 12g, Carbs 7.6g, Protein 3.2g

Kiwi Coconut Smoothie

Prep time: 3 minutes/ Cook time: 0 minutes / Serves 1

Ingredients
- 2 kiwis, pulp scooped
- 1 tbsp xylitol
- 4 ice cubes
- 2 cups unsweetened coconut milk
- 1 cup coconut yogurt
- Mint leaves to garnish

Directions:
1. Process the kiwis, xylitol, coconut milk, yogurt, and ice cubes in a blender, until smooth, for about 3 minutes. Transfer to serving glasses, garnish with mint leaves, and serve.

Nutritional information:
Calories 423, Fat 35.7g, Net Carbs 9.2g, Protein 14g

Mixed Nuts & Smoothie Breakfast

Prep time: 5 minutes/ Cook time: 0 minutes / Serves 2

Ingredients
- 3 cups buttermilk
- 2 tbsp peanut butter
- 1 tbsp unsweetened cocoa powder
- 2 tsp erythritol
- 1 cup mixed nuts, chopped for topping

Directions:
2. Combine the buttermilk, peanut butter, cocoa powder, and erythritol in a smoothie maker; puree until smooth and well mixed.
3. Share the smoothie into breakfast bowls, top with mixed nuts, and serve.

Nutritional information Calories 654, Fat 55.2g, Net Carbs 4.2g, Protein 16g

Superfood Red Smoothie

Prep time: 6 minutes/ Cook time: 0 minutes / Serves 1

Ingredients
- 1 Granny Smith apple, peeled and chopped
- 1 cup strawberries + extra for garnishing
- 1 cup blueberries
- 2 small beets, peeled and chopped
- 2/3 cup ice cubes
- ½ lemon, juiced
- 2 cups almond milk

Directions:
1. For the strawberries for garnishing, make a single deep cut on their sides, and set aside. In a smoothie maker, add the apples, strawberries, blueberries, beets, almond milk, and ice and blend the ingredients at high speed until nice and smooth, for about 75 seconds.
2. Add the lemon juice, and puree further for 30 seconds. Pour the drink into tall smoothie glasses, fix the reserved strawberries on each glass rim and serve with a straw.

Nutritional information:
Calories 233, Fat 4.3g, Carbs 11.3g, Protein 5g

Coconut Shake with Avocado

Prep time: 4 minutes/ Cook time: 0 minutes / Serves 2

Ingredients
- 3 cups coconut milk, chilled
- 1 avocado, pitted, peeled, sliced
- 2 tbsp erythritol
- Coconut cream for topping

Directions
1. Combine the coconut milk, avocado, and erythritol, into the smoothie maker, and blend for 1 minute to smooth.
2. Pour the drink into serving glasses, lightly add some coconut cream on top of them, and garnish with mint leaves. Serve immediately.

Nutritional information:
Calories 395, Fat: 27g, Carbs: 3.4g, Protein: 13.7g

Breakfast Cheesy Sausage

Prep time: 20 minutes/ Cook time: 5 minutes / Serves 1
Ingredients:
- 1 pork sausage link, cut open and casing discarded
- Sea salt and black pepper, to taste
- ½ teaspoon thyme
- ½ teaspoon sage
- ½ cup mozzarella cheese, shredded

Directions:
1. Mix sausage meat with thyme, sage, mozzarella cheese, sea salt and black pepper.
2. Shape the mixture into 2 equal-sized patties and transfer to a hot pan.
3. Cook for about 5 minutes per side and dish out to serve.

Nutritional information:
Calories 245, Carbs 0.8 g, Fats 19.6 g, Protein 15.7 g

Ham and Cheese Pockets

Prep time: 30 minutes/ Cook time: 20 minutes / Serves 1

Ingredients:
- 3 oz cream cheese
- 1 cup mozzarella cheese, shredded
- 3 tablespoons flax meal
- 4 oz provolone cheese slices
- 6 oz ham

Directions:
1. Preheat the oven to 400°F and line a baking sheet with parchment paper.
2. Microwave mozzarella cheese and cream cheese for about 1 minute.
3. Stir in the flax meal and combine well to make the dough.
4. Roll the dough and add provolone cheese slices and ham.
5. Fold the dough like an envelope, seal it and poke some holes in it.
6. Place on the baking sheet and transfer to the oven.
7. Bake for about 20 minutes until golden brown and remove from the oven.
8. Allow it to cool and cut in half while still hot to serve.

Nutritional information:
Calories 361, Carbs 7.9 g, Fats 27.6 g, Protein 24.8 g

Clementine and Pistachio Ricotta

Prep time: 10 minutes/ Cook time: 0 minutes / Serves 1

Ingredients:
- 3 teaspoons pistachios, chopped
- 1 cup ricotta
- 6 strawberries
- 2 tablespoon butter, melted
- 3 clementine, peeled and segmented

Directions:
1. Divide the ricotta into 2 serving bowls.
2. Top with clementine segments, strawberries, pistachios and butter to serve.

Nutritional information:
Calories 311, Carbs 12.7 g, Fats 25.1 g, Protein 10.7 g

Gingerbread-Spiced Breakfast Smoothie

Prep time: 2 minutes/ Cook time: 0 minutes / Serves 1

Ingredients:
- 1 cup Coconut Milk
- 1 bag Tea
- ¼ tsp Cinnamon Powder
- 1/8 tsp Nutmeg Powder
- 1/8 tsp Powdered Cloves
- 1/3 cup Chia Seeds
- 2 tbsp Flax Seeds

Directions:
1. Place the teabag in a cup and pour in hot water. Allow to steep for a few minutes.
2. Pour the tea into a blender together with the rest of the ingredients. Process until smooth.

Nutritional information:
Calories 649, Carbs 10 g, Fats 46 g, Protein 6 g

Vegan Breakfast Muffins

Prep time: 5 minutes/ Cook time: 3 minutes / Serves 1

Ingredients:
- 2 tbsp Almond Flour
- ½ tsp Baking Powder
- ½ tsp Salt
- 2 tbsp Ground Flax Seeds
- ¼ cup Coconut Milk
- 3 tbsp Avocado Oil

Directions:
1. Whisk together almond flour, ground flax, baking powder, and salt in a bowl.
2. Stir in coconut milk
3. Heat avocado oil in a non-stick pan.
4. Ladle in the batter and cook for 2-3 minutes per side.

Nutritional information:
Calories 194, Carbs 2 g, Fats 21 g, Protein 1 g

Vegan Breakfast Biscuits

Prep time: 10 minutes/ Cook time: 10 minutes / Serves 2

Ingredients:
- 1.5 cups Almond Flour
- 1 tbsp Baking Powder
- ¼ tsp Salt
- ½ tsp Onion Powder
- ½ cup Coconut Milk
- ¼ cup Nutritional Yeast
- 2 tbsp Ground Flax Seeds
- ¼ cup Olive Oil

Directions:
1. Preheat oven to 450ºF.
2. Whisk together all ingredients in a bowl.
3. Divide the batter into a pre-greased muffin tin.
4. Bake for 10 minutes.

Nutritional information:
Calories 406, Carbs 10 g, Fats 28 g, Protein 7 g

Vegan Breakfast Sausages

Prep time: 15 minutes/ Cook time: 12 minutes / Serves 2

Ingredients:
- 200 grams Portobella Mushrooms
- 150 grams Walnuts
- 1 tbsp Tomato Paste
- 75 grams Panko
- 1 tsp Paprika
- 1 tsp Dried Sage
- 1 tsp Salt
- ½ tsp Black Pepper

Directions:
1. Blend all ingredients in a food processor.
2. Divide mixture into serving-sized portions and shape into sausages.
3. Bake for 12 minutes at 375°F.
4. Serve.

Nutritional information:
Calories 371, Carbs 9 g, Fats 25 g, Protein 7 g

Quick Breakfast Yogurt

Prep time: 2 minutes/ Cook time: 8 minutes / Serves 2
Ingredients:
- 4 cups Full-Fat Coconut Milk
- 2 tbsp Coconut Milk Powder
- 100 grams Strawberries, for serving

Directions:
1. Whisk together coconut milk and milk powder in a microwave-safe bowl.
2. Heat on high for 8-9 minutes.
3. Top with fresh strawberries and choice of sweetener to serve.

Nutritional information:
Calories 186, Carbs 10 g, Fats 38 g, Protein 4 g

CHAPTER 2: LUNCH

Cheesy Spinach

Prep time: 15 minutes/ Cook time: 15 minutes / Serves 2

Ingredients:
- 1 tablespoon unsalted butter
- 1 small yellow onion, chopped
- ½ cup cream cheese, softened
- 1 (10-ounce) package frozen spinach, thawed and squeezed dry
- 2 tablespoons water
- Salt and ground black pepper, as required
- 1 teaspoon fresh lemon juice

Directions:
1. In a skillet, melt the butter over medium heat and sauté the onion for about 6-8 minutes.
2. Add the cream cheese and cook for about 2 minutes till melted completely.
3. Stir in the spinach and water and cook for about 4-5 minutes.
4. Stir in the salt, black pepper and lemon juice and remove from the heat.
5. Serve immediately.

Nutritional information:
Calories 301, Fat 26.6 g, Carbs 10 g, Protein 8.9 g

Creamy Brussels Sprout

Prep time: 15 minutes/ Cook time: 15 minutes / Serves 1

Ingredients:
- ¾ cup fresh Brussels sprouts, trimmed and halved
- 1 garlic clove, minced
- 1 tablespoon butter, melted
- 1 tablespoon Dijon mustard
- ¼ cup heavy whipping cream
- Salt and ground white pepper, as required

Directions:
1. Preheat the oven to 450 degrees F.
2. In a roasting pan, add the Brussels sprouts, garlic and butter and toss to coat well.
3. Roast for about 10-15 minutes, tossing occasionally.
4. Meanwhile, in a small pan, add the remaining ingredients over medium-low heat and bring to a gentle boil.
5. Cook for about 1-2 minutes, stirring continuously.
6. Serve Brussels sprouts with the topping of creamy sauce.

Nutritional information:
Calories 125, Fat 11.8 g, Carbs 3.6 g, Protein 1.6 g

Broccoli Stir Fry

Prep time: 10 minutes/ Cook time: 15 minutes / Serves 1

Ingredients:
- 1 tablespoon coconut oil
- 2 cups broccoli florets
- 1 tablespoon low-sodium soy sauce
- ¼ teaspoon garlic powder
- Ground black pepper, as required

Directions:
1. In a large pan, melt the coconut oil over medium heat and stir in the broccoli.
2. Cover the pan and cook for 10 minutes, stirring occasionally.
3. Stir in the soy sauce and spices and cook for about 5 minutes.
4. Serve hot.

Nutritional information:
Calories 93, Fat 7.1 g, Carbs 6.8 g, Protein 3.1 g

Beef Roast

Prep time: 10 minutes/ Cook time: 5 hours / Serves 2

Ingredients:
- 2 1/2 lbs. beef roast
- 1 tbsp ground coriander
- 1 tbsp garam masala
- 1 Serrano pepper, minced
- 1 tbsp ginger, grated
- 5 garlic cloves, minced
- 2 tbsp fresh lemon juice
- 20 curry leaves
- 1 tsp mustard seeds
- 2 tbsp coconut oil
- 1 large onion, chopped
- 1/4 cup coconut slices
- 1/2 tsp ground pepper
- 1 tsp turmeric
- 1 1/2 tsp chili powder
- 1 tsp salt

Directions:
1. Add oil, mustard seeds, onion, and salt into the crock pot and cook on high for 1 hour.
2. Add remaining ingredients except for coconut and cook on high for 3 hours.
3. Shred meat using a fork.
4. Add coconut slices and cook on high for 1 hour.
5. Serve and enjoy.

Nutritional information:
Calories 445, Fat 19 g, Carbs 7 g, Protein 59 g

Almond Cinnamon Beef Meatballs

Prep time: 10 minutes/ Cook time: 25 minutes / Serves 2

Ingredients:

- 2 lbs. ground beef
- 3 eggs
- ½ cup fresh parsley, minced
- 1 tsp cinnamon
- 1 ½ tsp dried oregano
- 2 tsp cumin
- 1 tsp garlic, minced
- 1 cup almond flour
- 1 medium onion, grated
- 1 tsp pepper
- 2 tsp salt

Directions:
1. Preheat the oven to 400 F.
2. Add all ingredients into the mixing bowl and mix until well combined.
3. Make small meatballs from mixture and place on greased baking tray and bake for 20-25 minutes.
4. Serve and enjoy.

Nutritional information:
Calories 325, Fat 16 g, Carbs 6 g, Protein 40 g

roganoff

minutes/ Cook time: 20 minutes / Serves 2

ics:
- 1 lb. beef strips
- 3/4 cup mushrooms, sliced
- 1 small onion, chopped
- 1 tbsp butter
- 2 tbsp olive oil
- 2 tbsp green onion, chopped
- 1/4 cup sour cream
- 1 cup chicken broth
- Pepper
- Salt

Directions:
1. Add meat in bowl and coat with 1 teaspoon oil, pepper and salt.
2. Heat remaining oil in a pan.
3. Add meat to pan and cook until golden brown on both sides.
4. Transfer meat in bowl and set aside.
5. Add butter in same pan.
6. Add onion and cook until onion softened.
7. Add mushrooms and sauté until the liquid is absorbed.
8. Add broth and cook until sauce thickened.
9. Add sour cream, green onion, and meat and stir well.
10. Cook over medium-high heat for 3-4 minutes.
11. Serve and enjoy.

Nutritional information:
Calories 345, Fat 20 g, Carbs 3 g, Protein 35 g

Baked Chicken Fajitas

Prep time: 10 minutes/ Cook time: 18 minutes / Serves 2

Ingredients:
- 1 1/2 lbs. chicken tenders
- 2 tbsp fajita seasoning
- 2 tbsp olive oil
- 1 onion, sliced
- 2 bell pepper, sliced
- 1 lime juice
- 1 tsp kosher salt

Directions:
1. Preheat the oven to 400 F.
2. Add all ingredients in a large mixing bowl and toss well.
3. Transfer bowl mixture on a baking tray and bake in preheated oven for 15-18 minutes.
4. Serve and enjoy.

Nutritional information:
Calories 286, Carbs 6.8 g, Fat 13 g, Protein 33 g

Baked Chicken Wings

Prep time: 10 minutes/ Cook time: 50 minutes / Serves 2

Ingredients:
- 2 lbs. chicken wings
- 1 tbsp. lemon pepper seasoning
- 2 tbsp butter, melted
- 4 tbsp olive oil

Directions:
1. Preheat the oven to 400 F.
2. Toss chicken wings with olive oil.
3. Arrange chicken wings on a baking tray and bake for 50 minutes.
4. In a small bowl, mix together lemon pepper seasoning and butter.
5. Remove wings from oven and brush with butter and seasoning mixture.
6. Serve and enjoy.

Nutritional information:

Calories 606, Fat 36 g, Carbs 1 g, Protein 65 g

Chicken with Spinach Broccoli

Prep time: 10 minutes/ Cook time: 10 minutes / Serves 2

Ingredients:
- 1 lb. chicken breasts, cut into pieces
- 4 oz cream cheese
- 1/2 cup parmesan cheese, shredded
- 2 cups baby spinach
- 2 cup broccoli florets
- 1 tomato, chopped
- 2 garlic cloves, minced
- 1 tsp Italian seasoning
- 2 tbsp olive oil
- Pepper
- Salt

Directions:
1. Heat oil in a saucepan over medium-high heat.
2. Add chicken, season with pepper, Italian seasoning, and salt and sauté for 5 minutes or until chicken cooked through.
3. Add garlic and sauté for a minute.
4. Add cream cheese, parmesan cheese, spinach, broccoli, and tomato and cook for 3-4 minutes more.
5. Serve and enjoy.

Nutritional information:
Calories 444, Fat 28 g, Carbs 5.9 g, Protein 40 g

Delicious Bacon Chicken

Prep time: 10 minutes/ Cook time: 40 minutes / Serves 2

Ingredients:
- 1 1/2 lbs. chicken breasts, cut in half
- 4 oz cheddar cheese, shredded
- 1/2 lb. bacon, cut into strips
- 1/2 tsp paprika
- 1/2 tsp onion powder
- 1/2 tsp garlic powder
- Pepper
- Salt

Directions:
1. Preheat the oven to 400 F.
2. In a small bowl, mix together paprika, onion powder, garlic powder, pepper, and salt.
3. Rub chicken with spice mixture.
4. Place chicken on a baking tray and top each with bacon piece.
5. Bake for 30 minutes. Remove from oven and sprinkle with cheese and bake for 10 minutes more.
6. Serve and enjoy.

Nutritional information:
Calories 642, Fat 36 g, Carbs 1.2 g, Protein 73 g

Mexican Chicken

Prep time: 10 minutes/ Cook time: 25 minutes / Serves 2

Ingredients:
- 2 cups chicken, cooked and shredded
- 1/2 cup Monterey jack cheese
- 1 1/2 cup cheddar cheese
- 3/4 cup chicken broth
- 2 tsp taco seasoning
- 12 oz cauliflower rice
- 14 oz Rotel tomatoes
- 2 garlic cloves, minced
- 1/3 cup green pepper, diced
- 1 onion, diced
- 1 tbsp butter

Directions:
1. Melt butter in a pan over medium heat.
2. Add garlic, pepper, and onion and sauté until softened.
3. Steam cauliflower rice according to packet instructions.
4. Add seasoning, broth, cauliflower rice, and Rotel to the pan.
5. Stir well and cook for 10 minutes.
6. Add chicken and cook for 5 minutes.
7. Top with cheese and cook until cheese is melted.
8. Serve and enjoy.

Nutritional information:
Calories 270, Fat 15 g, Carbs 8.1 g, Protein 24 g

Beef Casserole

Prep time: 10 minutes/ Cook time: 35 minutes / Serves 2

Ingredients:
- 1 lb. ground beef
- ½ cup mozzarella cheese, shredded
- ½ cup cheddar cheese, shredded
- 2 cans green beans, drained
- ½ tsp garlic powder
- ½ cup heavy cream
- ½ cup chicken broth
- 3 oz cream cheese
- ½ tsp pepper
- ½ tsp salt

Directions:
1. Preheat the oven to 350 F.
2. Brown meat in pan. Add cream cheese and stir until cheese is melted.
3. Add broth, garlic powder, heavy cream, pepper, and salt and stir well. Bring to boil.
4. Turn heat to medium and simmer until mixture thickened.
5. Add green beans then sprinkle cheese on top and bake in preheated oven for 25 minutes.
6. Serve and enjoy.

Nutritional information:
Calories 280, Carbs 4 g, Fat 20 g, Protein 18 g

Kelp noodle salad

Prep time: 10 minutes/ Cook time: 0 minutes / Serves 2
Salad Ingredients;
- 3 green onions, sliced
- 1 pack kelp noodles
- 1 cucumber, julienned
- ¼ cup carrots, grated
- ½ cup cashews, crushed
- 0.5 oz. cilantro, minced

Dressing ingredients;
- 2.3oz almond butter
- 1 garlic clove, minced
- 1 tablespoon tamari/ coconut aminos
- 1 tablespoon swerve
- 2 tablespoons lime juice
- 1 teaspoon chili oil/ chili infused extra-virgin olive oil
- 1 teaspoon ginger root, grated
- 1 teaspoon sesame oil
- Red pepper flakes, pinch
- Sea salt, pinch.

Directions:
1. In a bowl mix the salad ingredients.
2. In a jar, mix the dressing ingredients. (seal the jar and shake to mix well)
3. Pour the dressing into the initial bowl.
4. Toss to mix and serve.

Nutritional information:
Calories 240, Carbs 4.6 g, Fat 11 g, Protein 7 g

Spicy Satay Tofu Salad

Prep time: 8 minutes/ Cook time: 18 minutes / Serves 2
Ingredients:
- 1 (12 oz. pack) extra-firm tofu, drained and cubed
- ¼ cup peanut butter

- ½ tbsp. smoked paprika
- 1 tbsp. sesame oil
- ¼ tbsp. red chili flakes
- 2 drops liquid smoke
- 2 tbsp. water
- 1 tbsp. black sesame seeds

Salad:
- 4 cups fresh baby spinach leaves, rinsed, drained
- ¼ cup fresh mint leaves, chopped
- 2 tbsp. lemon juice
- 2 tbsp. avocado oil
- ¼ cup roasted cashews, unsalted

Directions:
1. Preheat oven to 395°F and use a parchment paper to line a baking tray.
2. Put the peanut butter, paprika, sesame oil, chili flakes, and liquid smoke into a large bowl.
3. Add the water to the bowl and mix thoroughly until all the ingredients are combined.
4. Put the tofu cubes in the bowl with the peanut butter mixture and stir gently until all cubes are evenly covered.
5. Transfer the covered tofu cubes onto the baking tray, spread them out evenly, and sprinkle the sesame seeds over them.
6. Bake the tofu cubes in the oven for about 20 minutes, or until browned and firm.
7. In a bowl, mix the salad ingredients together.
8. Take the tofu out of the oven and let the cubes cool for about 2 minutes.
9. Divide the salad and serve the tofu on top enjoy!

Nutritional information:
Calories 656.1, Carbs 5 g, Fats 54.4 g, Protein 29 g

Mexican Beef with Zucchini

Prep time: 10 minutes/ Cook time: 25 minutes / Serves 2

Ingredients:
- 1 ½ lbs. ground beef
- ¼ tsp red pepper flakes
- ½ tsp onion powder
- ½ tsp ground cumin
- ½ tbsp chili powder
- 10 oz salsa
- 2 garlic cloves, minced
- 2 zucchinis, diced
- ½ tsp pepper
- 1 tsp salt

Directions:
1. Brown meat in pan with garlic, pepper, and salt.
2. Add tomatoes and spices and stir well.
3. Cover and simmer over low heat for 10 minutes.
4. Add remaining ingredients and cook for 10 minutes more.
5. Serve and enjoy.

Nutritional information:
Calories 239, Fat 7.5 g, Carbs 6.2 g, Protein 36 g

Mexican Beef

Prep time: 10 minutes/ Cook time: 9 hours / Serves 2

Ingredients:
- 3 lbs. beef chuck roast
- ½ tsp red chili flakes
- 1 teaspoon oregano, dried
- ½ teaspoon paprika
- 1 teaspoon cumin
- 1 tbsp chili powder
- 2 tbsp lemon juice
- 2 tbsp tomato paste
- 3 garlic cloves, minced
- 1 onion, diced
- 1 tsp kosher salt

Directions:
1. In a small bowl, mix together all spices and set aside.
2. Add onion, garlic, lemon juice, and tomato paste in slow cooker and stir well.
3. Place meat into the slow cooker and sprinkle spice mixture all over meat.
4. Now cover and leave to cook on low for 8 hours.
5. Remove the meat from slow cooker and shred using fork.
6. Return shredded meat to the slow cooker and cook for 60 minutes more.
7. Serve and enjoy.

Nutritional information:
Calories 507, Fat 38 g, Carbs 2.7 g, Protein 36 g

7 minute noodles

Prep time: 2 minutes/ Cook time: 5 minutes / Serves 1

Ingredients:
- 1 oz. cream cheese
- 2 eggs
- ¼ tsp wheat gluten

Directions:
1. Preheat the oven to 325°F.
2. Mix the cream cheese, eggs, and wheat gluten until smooth.
3. Pour the mixture on a silicone mat on top of a heavy baking pan.
4. Spread out into a rectangle.
5. Bake for 5 minutes.
6. Remove from the oven and let it cool slightly.
7. Use a pizza wheel to cut into noodles.

Nutritional Information:
Calories 332, Carbs 0.6g, Fiber 2g, Fat 7.4g

Cheese head gnocchi

Prep time: 3 minutes/ Cook time: 3 minutes / Serves 2
Ingredients:
- 2 cups almond flour
- 2 cups mozzarella cheese, shredded
- ¼ cup butter
- 1 egg
- 1 egg yolk

Directions:
1. In a microwave safe dish, mix the cheese and butter and microwave for 2 minutes.
2. Mix and microwave for another minute.
3. Mix well until they're fully combined and let it cool slightly.
4. Add the egg, the egg yolk, and the almond flour.
5. Mix until a dough is formed.
6. Knead until the dough is semi-stretchy.
7. Roll the dough into a log that is 1 inch in diameter.
8. Cut small pieces and shape into disks.
9. Freeze the formed gnocchi in the freezer for 15 minutes.
10. Boil a pot of water and add a pinch of salt.
11. Add the frozen gnocchi and boil for 1-2 minutes until they're floating.
12. Cool for 5 minutes before adding any sauce.

Nutritional Information:
Calories 305, Carbs 6g, Fat 32g, Protein 25.8g

Fettuccine

Prep time: 5 minutes/ Cook time: 4 minutes / Serves 2

Ingredients:
- 3 tbsps. coconut flour
- 1 cup almond flour
- 2 tbsp. xanthan gum
- 1 egg
- ¼ tsp sea salt
- 2 tsp apple cider vinegar
- 3 tsp water
- 2 tbsps. butter
- ¼ cup heavy cream
- 2 cloves garlic
- 1 tbsp. parmesan cheese
- 1 tsp lemon zest
- salt and pepper

Directions:
1. Mix the coconut flour, almond flour, xanthan gum, egg, sea salt, apple cider vinegar, and water together.
2. Form the dough into a ball.
3. Cover with cling film and let it rest in the fridge for about 30 minutes.
4. Using a rolling pin, flatten the dough until it is about half an inch thick.
5. Use a pizza wheel to cut the dough into the shape of fettuccine.
6. Let the shaped pasta rest in the fridge for another 15 minutes.
7. Add the butter in a saucepan and let it brown. After, add the cream, garlic, lemon zest, and parmesan.
8. Add salt and pepper to taste.
9. Once the cheese is melted, add the pasta.
10. Cook until the pasta is cooked.

Nutritional Information:
Calories 353, Carbs 7g, Fat 23g, Protein 14g

Roasted Onions and Green Beans

Prep time: 10 minutes/ Cook time: 15 minutes / Serves 1

Ingredients:
- 1 yellow onion, sliced into rings
- ½ teaspoon onion powder
- 2 tablespoons coconut flour
- 1 1/3 cups fresh green beans, trimmed and chopped

Directions:
1. Take a large bowl and mix sunflower seeds with onion powder and coconut flour.
2. Add onion rings.
3. Mix well to coat.
4. Spread the rings in the baking sheet, lined with parchment paper.
5. Drizzle with some oil.
6. Bake for 10 minutes at 400 degrees F.
7. Parboil the green beans for 3 to 5 minutes in the boiling water.
8. Drain and serve the beans with baked onion rings.
9. Serve warm and enjoy!

Nutritional information:
Calories: 214, Carbs:3.7g, Fat: 19.4g, Protein: 8.3g

Roasted Green Beans

Prep time: 10 minutes/ Cook time: 20 minutes / Serves 4

Ingredients:
- 1 whole egg
- 2 tablespoons olive oil
- Sunflower seeds and pepper to taste
- 1 cup fresh green beans
- 5 ½ tablespoons grated parmesan cheese

Directions:
1. Pre-heat your oven to 400 degrees F.
2. Take a bowl and whisk in eggs with oil and spices.
3. Add beans and mix well.
4. Stir in parmesan cheese and pour the mix into baking pan (lined with parchment paper.
5. Bake for 15-20 minutes. Serve warm and enjoy!

Nutritional information:
Calories: 216, Carbs: 7g, Fat: 21g, Protein: 9g

Buttery Lamb Chops

Prep time: 10 minutes/ Cook time: 10 minutes / Serves 2

Ingredients:
- 1 lb. lamb chops
- 2 garlic cloves, minced
- 2 tbsp fresh basil, chopped
- 1/2 tsp garlic powder
- 2 tbsp butter
- 1 1/2 tsp Dijon mustard
- 1 tbsp olive oil

Directions:
1. Season pork chops with garlic powder and brush with oil.
2. Heat grill over medium-high heat.
3. Cook pork chops on hot grill for 4-5 minutes per side.
4. In a small bowl, mix together butter, mustard, and basil.
5. Spread butter mixture on each pork chops and serves.

Nutritional information:
Calories 295, Fat 17.6 g, Carbs 0.6 g, Protein 32.1 g

Lemon Herb Lamb Chops

Prep time: 10 minutes/ Cook time: 10 minutes / Serves

Ingredients:
- 1 1/2 lbs. lamb chops
- 1/4 cup olive oil
- 1/4 tsp pepper
- 1 1/2 tsp oregano
- 1 tsp thyme
- 2 garlic cloves, chopped
- 2 tbsp lemon juice
- 1/4 tsp salt

Directions:
1. Marinate the lamb chops in the mixture of garlic, oregano, thyme, lemon juice, olive oil, pepper, and salt. Cover and place in the fridge overnight.
2. Cook pork chops over a hot grill for 3-5 minutes per side.
3. Serve and enjoy.

Nutritional information:
Calories 435, Fat 24 g, Carbs 2 g, Protein 48 g

Fennel Grill Pork Chops

Prep time: 10 minutes/ Cook time: 10 minutes / Serves 4

Ingredients:
- 4 pork chops, bone-in
- 1 ¾ tsp dried sage, crumbled
- 1 tsp fennel seed, crushed
- 1/2 tsp dried thyme
- 1 ½ tsp dried rosemary, crumbled
- 1/3 cup olive oil
- 1 bay leaf, crushed
- 1 1/2 tsp salt

Directions:
1. In a bowl, mix together sage, bay leaf, fennel seed, thyme, rosemary, and salt.
2. Rub pork chops with herb sage mixture and brush with olive oil and place in fridge for overnight.
3. Preheat the grill over medium heat.
4. Place marinated pork chops on the hot grill and cook for 4 minutes on each side.
5. Serve and enjoy.

Nutritional information:
Calories 404, Fat 37 g, Carbs 1 g, Protein 1.6 g

CHAPTER 3: DINNER

Cauliflower Rice

Prep time: 5 minutes/ Cook time: 6 minutes / Serves 2

Ingredients:
- 1 head grated cauliflower head
- 1 tablespoon coconut aminos
- 1 pinch of sunflower seeds
- 1 pinch of black pepper
- 1 tablespoon Garlic Powder
- 1 tablespoon Sesame Oil

Directions:
1. Add cauliflower to a food processor and grate it.
2. Take a pan and add sesame oil, let it heat up over medium heat.
3. Add grated cauliflower and pour coconut aminos.
4. Cook for 4-6 minutes.
5. Season and enjoy!

Nutritional Information:
Calories: 329, Carbs: 13g, Fat: 28g, Protein: 10g

Spinach & Cauliflower Soup

Prep time: 10 minutes/ Cook time: 12 minutes / Serves 4

Ingredients:
- 1 White onion, diced
- 1 Cauliflower head, chopped
- 2 Garlic cloves, diced
- 1 Bay leaf (crumbled)
- 5.3 oz. Watercress
- 7.1 oz. Fresh spinach
- 4 cups Vegetable stock
- 1 cup Coconut milk
- ¼ cup Coconut oil
- 1 teaspoon Salt
- Ground black pepper

Directions:
- Place the onion and garlic in a soup pot greased with some ghee over medium flame and lightly brown it.
- Add the cauliflower and bay leaf and cook for 5 minutes.
- Mix in the watercress and spinach and stir cook for 3 minutes.
- Pour in the stock and bring to boil, cooking until the cauliflower is tender-crisp.
- Mix in the coconut milk, salt and pepper.
- Remove from the flame and blend using an immersion blender.

Nutritional Information:
Calories 392, Fat 37.6 g, Carbs 9.7 g, Protein 4.9 g

Oriental red cabbage salad

Prep time: 5 minutes/ Cook time: 20 minutes / Serves 2

Ingredients:
- ¼ tsp ground black pepper
- 4¼ oz. butter
- 2 tbsp. fresh dill, chopped
- 1 tbsp. red wine vinegar
- 30 oz. red cabbage
- 1 tsp salt
- 1 cinnamon stick
- 1 orange, juice and zest

Directions:
1. In a mandolin slicer or a food processor, finely shred the cabbage.
2. Fry in butter on medium high for 10-15 minutes. Softly fry the cabbage until it becomes shiny and soft, but not too brown.
3. Add pepper and salt. Put in orange juice, vinegar, and cinnamon. Allow it to cook for 5 -10 minutes.
4. Finally, when serving or towards the end, top with zest and dill.

Nutritional Information:
Calories 310, Fat 11.6 g, Carbs 10.7 g, Protein 5.9 g

Broccoli salad with fresh dill

Prep time: 5 minutes/ Cook time: 12 minutes / Serves 2

Ingredients:
- ¾ cup fresh dill
- 1 lb. broccoli
- Salt and ground black pepper to taste
- 1 cup mayonnaise

Directions:
1. Mix all the **Ingredients** together in a bowl.

Nutritional Information:
Calories 252, Carbs 5.7 g, Fat 10.6 g, Protein 10 g

Stuffed Zucchini

Prep time: 5 minutes/ Cook time: 30 minutes / Serves 1

Ingredients:
- 1 large zucchini
- 2 tbsp. olive oil
- ¼ cup green onion, chopped
- 1 garlic clove, minced
- 1 cup fresh baby spinach leaves
- A handful of fresh rocket, chopped
- Sea salt and black pepper to taste
- ¼ cup vegan cheese
- Pinch of dried parsley

Directions:
1. Preheat oven to 380°F and use a parchment paper to line a baking tray.
2. Cut the zucchini in half lengthwise and scoop out most of the pulp.
3. Mash the zucchini pulp in a small bowl with a masher and set it aside.
4. Heat a skillet over medium heat and add half of the olive oil.
5. Add the zucchini pulp, chopped onion, and minced garlic to the skillet.
6. Stir continuously, cooking the **Ingredients** for up to 5 minutes before adding the baby spinach and rocket.
7. Stir for a few seconds, add salt and pepper to taste, and turn off the heat.
8. Add the vegan cheese and stir well to ensure all **Ingredients** are incorporated and the cheese has melted.
9. Scoop the mixture into the zucchini halves and transfer them onto the baking tray.
10. Cover the baking tray with aluminum foil and transfer it to the oven.
11. Bake the stuffed zucchini halves for 25 minutes. Then, turn off the oven, uncover the baking tray, and put the uncovered zucchini halves back into the oven for about

    5 minutes.
12. Serve the stuffed zucchini garnished with the remaining olive oil and some dried parsley.
13. Serve and enjoy!

Nutritional Information:
Calories 359.5, Carbs 7 g, Fats 32.5 g, Protein 7.3 g

Coconut pasta

Prep time: 3 minutes/ Cook time: 4 minutes / Serves 1

Ingredients:
- 1 egg
- 3 tbsps. glucomannan powder
- 3 tbsps. oat fiber
- ½ tsp kosher salt
- 1 tbsp. baking powder
- 2 tsp coconut flour
- 1 cups water

Directions:
- Mix the dry **Ingredients** in a large bowl.
- In a separate bowl, beat the egg until foamy.
- Add the egg on top of the dry **Ingredients** and mix until the mixture turns into a fine powder.
- Add the water and mix with your hands until the dough becomes smooth, yet sticky.
- Let the dough sit for 10 minutes.
- Run the dough through a pasta press using the spaghetti attachment or roll it out using a rolling pin and cut into 1/3-inch-wide ribbons.
- Boil some chicken broth and add the pasta in.
- Cook for 4 minutes and drain the broth.

Nutritional Information:
Calories 268, Carbs 5.1 g, Fat 0.7 g, Protein 0.9 g

Spinach pasta

Prep time: 2 minutes/ Cook time: 3 minutes / Serves 2

Ingredients:
- 3 oz. spinach
- 2 eggs
- ½ tsp salt
- 1 ½ tsp olive oil
- 2 cups almond flour
- ½ cup coconut flour, for kneading

Directions:
1. Cook the spinach on medium heat until it turns bright green.
2. Prepare an ice bath for the spinach by combining ice and water in a large bowl.
3. Remove the spinach from the skillet and submerge it in the ice water.
4. Once the spinach is lukewarm, drain and squeeze the extra water with a cloth.
5. Combine the spinach, eggs, salt, and olive oil in a bowl.
6. Mix until everything is smooth.
7. Slowly add the almond flour to make the dough.
8. Once the dough is formed, let it sit for 25 minutes.
9. Dust a flat workplace with a generous amount of coconut flour and knead the dough with it until the dough is no longer sticky. Add as needed.
10. Cut the dough into 4 pieces.
11. Roll each piece with a rolling pin.
12. Using a pizza wheel, cut 3-4 inch blocks out of the dough.
13. Cut the blocks in a zigzag motion to create medium sized triangles.
14. Once all of them are cut, dust the triangles with some coconut flour.
15. Take a piece of the triangle shaped pasta, wet your fingers and stick two of the ends together.
16. Repeat with all of the triangle pieces.

17. Lower the pasta gently in a pot of boiling water and cook for 3 minutes.
18. Remove each piece and transfer to a plate.

Nutritional Information:
Calories 165, Carbs 5 g, Fat 17 g, Protein 13.6 g

Avocado Fries

Prep time: 3 minutes/ Cook time: 25 minutes / Serves 1

Ingredients:
- 1 tbsp. olive oil
- ¼ cup almond flour
- ¼ tsp. cayenne pepper
- ¼ tsp. smoked paprika
- Pinch of salt
- ¾ tbsp. unsweetened almond milk
- 1 medium Hass avocado, pitted, peeled
- 1 tsp. lime juice

Directions:
1. Preheat the oven to 400°F.
2. Use a parchment paper to line a baking tray and grease the paper with olive oil.
3. In a small bowl, combine the flour, cayenne pepper, smoked paprika, and salt.
4. Pour the almond milk into another small bowl.
5. Slice the peeled avocado into 10 equally-sized fries.
6. Coat all sides of the fries in the flour mixture, dip in almond milk, and coat with another layer of flour.
7. Transfer the coated fries to the greased baking tray.
8. Bake the fries for 5 minutes, then flip them over and bake for another 10 minutes. Flip the fries again and bake for 5 more minutes.
9. Flip the fries one more time, sprinkle them with the lime juice, and bake them for a final 5 minutes.
10. Remove the baking tray out of the oven and allow the fries to cool down for a few minutes.
11. Serve warm with any low-carb (vegan) sauce and enjoy!

Nutritional Information:
Calories 333.7, Carbs 4 g, Fats 31.9 g, Protein 7 g

Mushroom Zoodle Pasta

Prep time: 10 minutes/ Cook time: 16 minutes / Serves 2

Ingredients:
- 3 large zucchinis
- ½ tsp. salt
- 1 tbsp. coconut oil
- 1 large green onion, diced
- 3 garlic cloves, minced
- 5 cups oyster mushrooms, chopped
- Pinch each of nutmeg, onion powder, paprika powder, white pepper, and salt
- 1 cup full-fat coconut milk
- ½ cup vegan mozzarella
- ½ cup baby spinach leaves, chopped
- ¼ cup fresh thyme, chopped
- 1 tbsp. miso paste

Directions:
1. In a large bowl, toss the zoodles or zucchini slices with half a teaspoon of salt and set aside.
2. Add coconut oil in a large skillet, over medium heat, and add the coconut oil.
3. Add the onion and cook until translucent, for about 5 minutes while stirring occasionally.
4. Stir in the minced garlic, chopped mushrooms, and remaining seasonings.
5. Cook all Ingredients in the skillet for about 3 minutes, stirring continuously.
6. Reduce heat to medium-low and slowly incorporate the coconut milk, followed by the mozzarella.
7. Cover the skillet and let the Ingredients heat through for about 8 minutes, stirring occasionally.
8. Drain any excess liquid from the salted zoodles by dabbing them with paper towels.
9. Add the dry zoodles to the skillet with the chopped spinach and stir well until all **Ingredients** are combined.
10. Turn off the heat and top the mushroom zoodle pasta with the chopped thyme.

11. Add more seasonings to taste, serve the pasta in a bowl, and enjoy!

Nutritional Information:
Calories 421.6, Carbs 13 g, Fats 34.9 g, Protein 11.5 g

Quick Veggie Protein Bowl

Prep time: 5 minutes/ Cook time: 13 minutes / Serves 1

Ingredients:
- 4 oz. extra-firm tofu, drained
- ¼ tsp. turmeric
- ¼ tsp. cayenne pepper
- 1 tbsp. coconut oil
- 1 cup broccoli florets, diced
- 1 cup Chinese kale, diced
- ½ cup button mushrooms, diced
- ½ tsp. dried oregano
- Himalayan salt
- Black pepper to taste
- ½ tsp. paprika
- ¼ cup of fresh oregano, diced

Directions:
1. Cut the tofu into tiny pieces and season with the turmeric and cayenne pepper.
2. Warm a large skillet and add ¾ of the coconut oil.
3. Once oil is heated, add the tofu and cook it for about 5 minutes, stirring continuously.
4. Transfer the cooked tofu to a medium-sized bowl and set it aside.
5. Add the remaining coconut oil, diced broccoli florets, Chinese kale, button mushrooms, and the remaining herbs to the skillet. Use paprika, pepper, and salt to taste.
6. Cook the vegetables for 6-8 minutes, stirring continuously.
7. Transfer the cooked veggies and tofu to the bowl. Garnish with the optional fresh oregano.
8. Serve and enjoy!

Nutritional Information:
Calories 596, Carbs 6 g, Fats 20.95 g, Protein 17.8 g

Tasty Green Salad

Prep time: 6 minutes/ Cook time: 0 minutes / Serves 2

Ingredients:
- 4 teaspoons white wine vinegar
- ½ cup cherry tomatoes, halved
- 2 teaspoons olive oil
- Dash pepper
- 1/8 teaspoon salt
- 2 teaspoons minced fresh basil
- 3 cups torn mixed salad greens
- ¾ teaspoon honey
- 1 tablespoon shredded Parmesan cheese

Directions:
1. Whisk vinegar, fresh basil, olive oil, honey, salt and dash pepper in a small bowl until blended.
2. In a separate large bowl combine tomatoes and salad greens.
3. Drizzle with vinaigrette and sprinkle with cheese.
4. Enjoy your meal.

Nutritional Information:

Calories:1092, Carbs: 15g, Fat: 86 g, Protein: 57 g

Asparagus and Artichoke Salad

Prep time: 15 minutes/ Cook time: 45 minutes / Serves 2

Ingredients:
- 20 tender, fresh green asparagus stalks (woody stem removed, rinsed)
- 8 fresh, medium artichokes
- 4 tablespoons extra virgin olive oil
- 2 cloves garlic, peeled and chopped
- 1 ounce chopped pistachio nuts
- 1 large egg white
- 4 teaspoons chopped green onions + 1 green onion for garnish, chopped
- Juice of 1 lemon
- Salt and white pepper to taste

Directions:
1. Fill a large pot ¾ of the way with water; add half the lemon juice and a generous sprinkle of salt.
2. Trim the artichokes by removing the leaves until you get to the light-yellow leaves. Set the hearts aside.
3. Place the artichoke leaves in boiling water. Cook 45 minutes. Once boiled, rinse under cold water.
4. Place the artichoke leaves in a food processor. Add the remaining lemon juice, half a glass of water (4 ounces), a pinch of salt and pepper, pistachios, green onions, garlic, and egg white. Blend for 1 minute. Add the olive oil slowly. Continue to blend until smooth.
5. Cut up the artichoke hearts and arrange on a plate. Place the asparagus over the top. Drizzle the sauce over the artichokes and asparagus. Garnish with fresh green onions. Serve.

Nutritional Information:
Calories 444, Carbs: 10g, Fat: 1g, Protein: 13g

Soy flour noodles

Prep time: 3 minutes/ Cook time: 2 minutes / Serves 2

Ingredients:
- 1 ½ cups soy flour
- ¾ cup gluten
- 2 tsp salt
- 2 tbsps. warm water
- 2 tsp olive oil

Directions:
1. Add the soy flour, gluten, and salt in a mixing bowl and mix well.
2. Add the rest of the **Ingredients** and form a dough ball.
3. Wrap in plastic film and rest in the fridge for half an hour to 45 minutes.
4. Cut the dough into 8 equal pieces and process through your pasta cutter or flatten the dough using a rolling pin on a flat surface and use a pizza wheel to cut into small noodles.
5. Bring a pot of water to boil.
6. Add a pinch of salt.
7. Cook the noodles for 2 minutes, drain the water and your noodles are ready.

Nutritional Information:
Calories 322, Carbs 5.2g, Fat 15g, Protein 41g

Shrimp Scampi

Prep time: 10 minutes/ Cook time: 25 minutes / Serves 2

Ingredients:
- 1 lb. shrimp, peeled and deveined
- 4 tbsp parmesan cheese, grated
- 1 cup chicken broth
- 1 tbsp garlic, minced
- ½ cup butter

Directions:
1. Preheat the oven to 350 F.
2. Melt butter in a saucepan over medium heat.
3. Add garlic and sauté for minute. Add broth and stir well.
4. Add shrimp to glass dish and pour butter mixture over shrimp.
5. Top with grated cheese and bake for 10-12 minutes.
6. Serve and enjoy.

Nutritional Information:
Calories 388, Fat 27 g, Carbs 2.7 g, Protein 30.4 g

Grilled Salmon
Prep time: 10 minutes/ Cook time: 25 minutes / Serves 2
Ingredients:
- 2 salmon fillets
- 1 tsp dried rosemary
- 2 garlic cloves, minced
- ¼ tsp pepper
- 1 tsp salt

Directions:
1. In a bowl, mix together rosemary, garlic, pepper, and salt.
2. Add salmon fillets in a bowl and coat well and let sit for 15 minutes.
3. Preheat the grill.
4. Place marinated salmon fillets on hot grill and cook for 10-12 minutes.
5. Serve and enjoy.

Nutritional Information:
Calories 240, Fat 11 g, Carbs 1 g, Protein 34 g

Shrimp and Garlic

Prep time: 5 minutes/ Cook time: 15 minutes / Serves 2

Ingredients:
- 1 lb. shrimp, peeled and deveined
- 1 tsp parsley, chopped
- 2 tbsp lemon juice
- 5 garlic cloves, minced
- 3 tbsp butter
- Salt

Directions:
1. Melt butter in a pan over high heat.
2. Add shrimp in pan and cook for 1 minutes. Season with salt.
3. Stir and cook shrimp until turn to pink.
4. Add lemon juice and garlic and cook for 2 minutes.
5. Turn heat to medium and cook for 4 minutes more.
6. Garnish with parsley and serve.

Nutritional Information:
Calories 219, Fat 10.6 g, Carbs 3.2 g, Protein 26 g

Salmon Patties

Prep time: 10 minutes/ Cook time: 10 minutes / Serves 2

Ingredients:

- 14.5 oz can salmon
- 4 tbsp butter
- 1 avocado, diced
- 2 eggs, lightly beaten
- ½ cup almond flour
- ½ onion, minced
- Pepper
- Salt

Directions:

1. Add all **Ingredients** except butter in a large mixing bowl and mix until well combined.
2. Make six patties from mixture. Set aside.
3. Melt butter in a pan over medium heat.
4. Place patties on pan and cook for 4-5 minutes on each side.
5. Serve and enjoy.

Nutritional Information:

Calories 619, Fat 49 g, Carbs 11 g, Protein 36 g

Beef Stew

Prep time: 10 minutes/ Cook time: 55 minutes / Serves 2

Ingredients:
- 1 lb. flank steak, cut into chunks
- 1 Tablespoon olive oil
- 1 Tablespoon thyme
- 1 Tablespoon salt
- 4 cups beef stock
- 2 Tablespoons butter
- 1 carrot, chopped
- 2 stalks celery, chopped
- 1 14.5 oz can dice tomatoes
- ¼ onion, chopped
- 2 cloves garlic, minced
- 2 Tablespoons Worcestershire sauce
- ½ cup red wine (optional)
- 1 cup heavy cream

Directions:
1. Preheat a large pot over medium heat. Drizzle the oil, and brown the beef on all sides- about 4 minutes. Remove from pan and set aside.
2. In the same pot, melt in the butter and sauté the vegetables with the salt, until soft - about 3 minutes. Add in the herbs. Return the beef back to the pot.
3. Add the stock and Worcestershire sauce and wine. Bring to a boil, then reduce heat to low. Simmer 25 minutes. Stir in the cream, and simmer another 15 minutes. You could also make this in a crockpot!
4. After browning the beef, add the rest of the **Ingredients** (except cream) to the crockpot and cook on low 4-6 hours.
5. Turn heat off, let sit for 30 minutes to cool down, then add the heavy cream.

Nutritional Information:
Calories 450, Carbs 4.5 g, Fats 30.4 g, Proteins 35 g

CHAPTER 4: SNACKS

Coconut Cheesecake
Prep time: 10 minutes/ Cook time: 25 minutes / Serves 2
Ingredients
Crust:
- 2 egg whites
- ¼ cup erythritol
- 3 cups desiccated coconut
- 1 tsp coconut oil
- ¼ cup melted butter

Filling:
- 3 tbsp lemon juice
- 6 ounces raspberries
- 2 cups erythritol
- 1 cup whipped cream
- Zest of 1 lemon
- 24 ounces cream cheese

Directions:
1. Grease bottom and sides of a springform pan with coconut oil. Line with parchment paper. Preheat oven to 350ºF and mix all crust **Ingredients**. Pour the crust into the pan. Bake for about 25 minutes; let cool.
2. Meanwhile, beat the cream cheese with an electric mixer until soft. Add the lemon juice, zest, and erythritol. Fold the whipped cream into the cheese cream mixture. Fold in the raspberries gently. Spoon the filling into the baked and cooled crust. Place in the fridge for 4 hours.

Nutritional Information:
Calories 256, Fats 25 g, Carbs 3 g, Protein 5 g

Raspberry Nut Truffles
Prep time: 5 minutes/ Cook time: 4 minutes / Serves 2
Ingredients:
- 2 cups raw cashews
- 2 tbsp flax seed
- 1 ½ cups sugar-free raspberry preserves
- 3 tbsp swerve
- 10 oz unsweetened chocolate chips
- 3 tbsp olive oil

Directions:
1. Line a baking sheet with parchment paper and set aside. Grind the cashews and flax seeds in a blender for 45 seconds until smoothly crushed; add the raspberry and 2 tbsp of swerve.
2. Process further for 1 minute until well combined. Form 1-inch balls of the mixture, place on the baking sheet, and freeze for 1 hour or until firmed up.
3. Melt the chocolate chips, oil, and 1tbsp of swerve in a microwave for 1 ½ minutes. Toss the truffles to coat in the chocolate mixture, put on the baking sheet, and freeze further for at least 2 hours.

Nutritional Information:
Calories 251, Fats 18.3 g, Carbs 3.5 g, Protein 12 g

Chocolate Cakes

Prep time: 5 minutes/ Cook time: 20 minutes / Serves 2

Ingredients
- ½ cup almond flour
- ¼ cup xylitol
- 1 tsp baking powder
- ½ tsp baking soda
- 1 tsp cinnamon, ground
- A pinch of salt
- A pinch of ground cloves
- ½ cup butter, melted
- ½ cup buttermilk
- 1 egg
- 1 tsp pure almond extract

For the Frosting:
- 1 cup heavy cream
- 1 cup dark chocolate, flaked

Directions:
1. Start by preheating the oven to 360ºF. Use a cooking spray to grease a donut pan.
2. In a bowl, mix the cloves, almond flour, baking powder, salt, baking soda, xylitol, and cinnamon. In a separate bowl, combine the almond extract, butter, egg, and buttermilk. Mix the wet mixture into the dry mixture. Evenly ladle the batter into the donut pan. Bake for 17 minutes.
3. Set a pan over medium heat and warm heavy cream; simmer for 2 minutes. Fold in the chocolate flakes; combine until all the chocolate melts; let cool. Spread the top of the cakes with the frosting.

Nutritional Information:
Calories 218, Fats 20 g, Carbs 10 g, Protein 4.8 g

Blueberry Ice Pops
Prep time: 5 minutes/ Cook time: 0 minutes / Serves 2

Ingredients
- 3 cups blueberries
- ½ tbsp lemon juice
- ¼ cup swerve
- ¼ cup water

Directions:
1. Pour the blueberries, lemon juice, swerve, and water in a blender, and puree on high speed for 2 minutes until smooth. Strain through a sieve into a bowl, discard the solids.
2. Mix in more water if too thick. Divide the mixture into ice pop molds, insert stick cover, and freeze for 4 hours to 1 week. When ready to serve, dip in warm water and remove the pops.

Nutritional Information:
Calories 48, Fats 1.2 g, Carbs 7.9 g, Protein 2.3 g

Strawberry Vanilla Shake

Prep time: 2 minutes/ Cook time: 0 minutes / Serves 1

Ingredients
- 2 cups strawberries, stemmed and halved
- 12 strawberries to garnish
- ½ cup cold unsweetened almond milk
- 2/3 tsp vanilla extract
- ½ cup heavy whipping cream
- 2 tbsp swerve

Directions:
1. Process the strawberries, milk, vanilla extract, whipping cream, and swerve in a large blender for 2 minutes; work in two batches if needed The shake should be frosty.
2. Pour into glasses, stick in straws, garnish with strawberry halves, and serve.

Nutritional Information:
Calories 285, Fats 22.6 g, Carbs 3.1 g, Protein 16 g

Vanilla Ice Cream

Prep time: 5 minutes/ Cook time: 0 minutes / Serves 2

Ingredients
- ½ cup smooth peanut butter
- ½ cup swerve
- 3 cups half and half
- 1 tsp vanilla extract
- 2 pinches salt

Directions:
1. Beat peanut butter and swerve in a bowl with a hand mixer until smooth.
2. Gradually whisk in half and half until thoroughly combined. Mix in vanilla and salt.
3. Pour mixture into a loaf pan and freeze for 45 minutes until firmed up.
4. Scoop into glasses when ready to eat and serve.

Nutritional Information:
Calories 290, Fats 23 g, Carbs 6 g, Protein 13 g

Chia and Blackberry Pudding

Prep time: 10 minutes/ Cook time: 0 minutes / Serves 1

Ingredients
- 1/2 cup full-fat natural yogurt
- 2 tsp swerve
- 2 tbsp chia seeds
- 1 cup fresh blackberries
- 1 tbsp lemon zest
- Mint leaves, to serve

Directions:
1. Mix together the yogurt and the swerve. Stir in the chia seeds. Reserve 4 blackberries for garnish and mash the remaining ones with a fork until pureed. Stir in the yogurt mixture
2. Chill in the fridge for 30 minutes. When cooled, divide the mixture between 2 glasses.
3. Top each with a couple of blackberries, mint leaves, lemon zest and serve.

Nutritional Information:
Calories 169, Fats 10 g, Carbs 4.7 g, Protein 7.5 g

Almond Butter Fat Bombs

Prep time: 3 minutes/ Cook time: 0 minutes / Serves 2

Ingredients
- ½ cup almond butter
- ½ cup coconut oil
- 4 tbsp unsweetened cocoa powder
- ½ cup erythritol

Directions:
1. Melt butter and coconut oil in the microwave for 45 seconds, stirring twice until properly melted and mixed.
2. Mix in cocoa powder and erythritol until completely combined.
3. Pour into muffin molds and refrigerate for 3 hours to harden.

Nutritional Information:
Calories 193, Fats 18.3 g, Carbs 2 g, Protein 4 g

Mixed Berry Trifle

Prep time: 3 minutes/ Cook time: 0 minutes / Serves 2

Ingredients
- ½ cup walnuts, toasted
- 1 avocado, chopped
- 1/2 cup mascarpone cheese, softened
- 1/2 cup fresh blueberries
- 1/2 cup fresh raspberries
- 1/2 cup fresh blackberries

Directions:
1. In four dessert glasses, share half of the mascarpone, half of the berries (mixed), half of the walnuts, and half of the avocado, and repeat the layering process for a second time to finish the ingredients.
2. Cover the glasses with plastic wrap and refrigerate for 45 minutes until quite firm.

Nutritional Information:
Calories 321, Fats 28 g, Carbs 8.3 g, Protein 9.8 g

Walnut Cookies

Prep time: 7 minutes/ Cook time: 12 minutes / Serves 2

Ingredients
- 1 egg
- 2 cups ground pecans
- ¼ cup sweetener
- ½ tsp baking soda
- 1 tbsp butter
- 8 walnuts halves

Directions:
1. Preheat oven to 350ºF. Mix the ingredients, except the walnuts, until combined.
2. Make 8 balls out of the mixture and press them with your thumb onto a lined cookie sheet.
3. Top each cookie with a walnut half. Bake for about 12 minutes.

Nutritional Information:
Calories 101, Fats 11 g, Carbs 0.6 g, Protein 1.6 g

Cinnamon and Turmeric Latte

Prep time: 10 minutes/ Cook time: 5 minutes / Serves 2

Ingredients
- 2 cups almond milk
- ⅓ tsp cinnamon powder
- 1 cup brewed coffee
- ½ tsp turmeric powder
- 1 ½ tsp erythritol
- Cinnamon sticks to garnish

Directions:
1. In the blender, add the almond milk, cinnamon powder, coffee, turmeric, and erythritol. Blend the ingredients at medium speed for 45 seconds and pour the mixture into a saucepan.
2. Set the pan over low heat and heat through for 5 minutes; do not boil. Keep swirling the pan to prevent from boiling.
3. Turn the heat off, and serve in latte cups, with a cinnamon stick in each one.

Nutritional Information:
Calories 132, Fats 12 g, Carbs 0.3 g, Protein 3.9 g

Chocolate Bark with Almonds

Prep time: 5 minutes/ Cook time: 0 minutes / Serves 2

Ingredients
- ½ cup toasted almonds, chopped
- ½ cup butter
- 6 drops stevia
- ¼ tsp salt
- ½ cup unsweetened coconut flakes
- 2 ounces dark chocolate

Directions:
1. Melt together the butter and chocolate, in the microwave, for 90 seconds. Remove and stir in stevia.
2. Line a cookie sheet with waxed paper and spread the chocolate evenly. Scatter the almonds on top, coconut flakes, and sprinkle with salt.
3. Refrigerate for one hour.

Nutritional Information:
Calories 161, Fats 15.3 g, Carbs 1.9 g, Protein 1.9 g

Vanilla Berry Mug Cake

Prep time: 3 minutes/ Cook time: 1 minutes / Serves 1

Ingredients:
- 6 frozen raspberries
- 2 tbsp coconut flour
- ¼ tsp baking powder
- 1 tbsp butter, melted
- 1 egg medium
- 1 tbsp granulated sweetener
- 2 tbsp cream cheese
- 1 tsp vanilla extract

Directions:
1. Microwave the cream cheese and butter together in a mug on high for 20 seconds.
2. Add the baking powder, coconut flour, vanilla extract and granulated sweetener to the butter and cream cheese mixture. Mix until all the ingredients are combined.
3. Add the egg to the mixture and keep mixing until fully combined and smooth batter is prepared.
4. Add the frozen raspberries and press them gently from the top.
5. Place in the microwave and keep on high for 2 minutes.
6. Enjoy the amazing vanilla berry mug cake.

Nutritional Information:
Calories 330, Fat 14.5g, Carbohydrate 38.3g, Protein 11.5g

Pumpkin Spice Mug Cake

Prep time: 4 minutes/ Cook time: 1 minutes / Serves 1

Ingredients:
- 1 egg
- 2 tbsp almond meal
- 2 tsp granulated erythritol
- 2 tbsp butter
- 2 tsp pumpkin spice
- 1 tbsp coconut flour
- 1 tbsp heavy cream
- ¼ tsp baking powder

Directions:
1. Put butter in a microwave bowl and microwave it for half a minute or until melted.
2. Remove the bowl from the microwave once butter is melted.
3. Add coconut flour, baking powder, almond meal and pumpkin spice to the melted butter and mix until well combined.
4. Add egg, butter, heavy cream and erythritol to the mixture and keep mixing until fully combined.
5. Place the bowl again in the microwave to cook the mixture on high for a minute.
6. Remove from the microwave once cooked.
7. Transfer to the serving mug and enjoy the delicious, moist and fluffy pumpkin spice mug cake with heavy cream at the top.

Nutritional Information:
Calories 460, Fat 41.3g, Carbohydrate 22.3g, Protein 10.8g

Berry Acai Smoothie

Prep time: 2 minutes/ Cook time: 0 minutes / Serves 1

Ingredients:
- 1 cup Silk Tofu
- 2 tbsp Coconut Cream
- 1 cup Ice Cubes
- ¼ cup Raspberries
- 2 tbsp Acai Powder
- 3 tbsp Soy Protein Powder

Directions:
1. Combine all ingredients in a blender.
2. Blend until smooth.

Nutritional Information:
Calories 556, Carbs 10 g, Fats 20 g, Protein 18 g

Choco-Coco Milk Shake

Prep time: 5 minutes/ Cook time: 0 minutes / Serves 1

Ingredients:
- ½ cup whole milk
- 1 tbsp cocoa powder
- 1 packet Stevia, or more to taste
- 1 tbsp coconut flakes, unsweetened
- 1 cup water
- 1 tbsp coconut oil

Directions:
1. Add all ingredients in blender.
2. Blend until smooth and creamy.
3. Serve and enjoy.

Nutritional Information:
Calories 263, Carbs 22.7g, Proteins 4.8g, Fats 20.65g

Nutty Choco Milk Shake
Prep time: 5 minutes/ Cook time: 0 minutes / Serves 1
Ingredients:
- ¼ cup whole milk
- 1 tbsp cocoa powder
- 1 packet Stevia, or more to taste
- ¼ cup pecans
- 1 ½ cups water
- 1 tbsp macadamia oil

Directions:
1. Add all ingredients in blender.
2. Blend until smooth and creamy.
3. Serve and enjoy.

Nutritional Information:
Calories 358, Carbs 15.5g, Proteins 5.1g, Fats 34.0g

Choco Milk Smoothie
Prep time: 4 minutes/ Cook time: 0 minutes / Serves 1
Ingredients:
- ¼ cup whole milk
- 1 tbsp cocoa powder
- 1 packet Stevia, or more to taste
- 1 tbsp chia seeds
- 1 tbsp hemp seeds
- 1 tbsp flaxseed
- 1 ½ cups water
- 1 tbsp Flaxseed oil

Directions:
1. Add all ingredients in blender.
2. Blend until creamy yet still gritty. If preferred, blend until smooth.
3. Serve and enjoy.

Nutritional Information:
Calories 363, Carbs 22.8g, Proteins 8.9g, Fats 29.4g

Creamy Choco Shake
Prep time: 4 minutes/ Cook time: 0 minutes / Serves 1
Ingredients:
- ½ cup heavy cream
- 2 tbsps cocoa powder
- 1 packet Stevia, or more to taste
- 1 cup water

Directions:
1. Add all ingredients in blender.
2. Blend until smooth and creamy.
3. Serve and enjoy.

Nutritional Information:
Calories 435, Carbs 10.6g, Proteins 4.6g, Fats 45.5g

Baby Kale and Yogurt Smoothie

Prep time: 4 minutes/ Cook time: 0 minutes / Serves 1

Ingredients:
- 1 cup whole milk yogurt
- 1 cup baby kale greens
- 1 packet Stevia, or more to taste
- 1 tbsp MCT oil
- 1 tbsp sunflower seeds
- 1 cup water

Directions:
1. Add all ingredients in blender.
2. Blend until smooth and creamy.
3. Serve and enjoy.

Nutritional Information:
Calories 329, Carbs 15.6g, Proteins 11.0g, Fats 26.2g

Raspberry Chocolate Fudge

Prep time: 2 minutes/ Cook time: 10 minutes / Serves 2

Ingredients
- ¼ cup raw cacao powder
- 1 Tablespoon unsweetened dark chocolate, shaved
- 1 Tablespoon Stevia
- ¼ cup coconut oil
- ¼ cup raspberries, mashed lightly
- ¼ cup almond milk

Directions:
1. Mix all ingredients together until well combined. Prepare a 10" baking dish with parchment paper or plastic wrap, and carefully spoon the fudge mixture into the center.
2. Using a spatula, spread the mixture evenly into the baking dish, and cover with plastic wrap.
3. Refrigerate for an hour, and cut into 8 equal pieces. Store wrapped in the fridge for up to one month.

Nutritional Information:
Calories 74, Carbs 0.9 g, Fats 8.1 g, Proteins 0.6 g

CONCLUSION

Thank you for getting to the end of this book. I hope you've enjoyed reading and that you'll have fun replicating these recipes on your own. Keto can seem challenging at first as a single person, but once you get the hang of it, it will be worth the effort.

I am confident that you will make it through your lifestyle change and that you will feel all the better for the changes that will happen. From improved mental focus to better energy, and weight loss, there is almost no reason why you should not hop on the Keto train today!

Additional Resources

Free keto Macros Calculator

https://highkey.com/pages/keto-calculator2

Day after day I hear dozens of people voice the following problems (perhaps one or more of them apply to you.)

- I don't know how to figure out my macros.
- I can never keep straight how much protein, fat, or carbs I'm supposed to eat.
- Keto food is boring.
- Everyone else is losing weight on Keto but me.
- I lost some weight in the beginning but now I've stalled for a long time.

If any of the above applies to you, here is your answer. https://bit.ly/3iS4khx

Keto Breads

Great New! You Don`t Have To Give Up Your Favorite Bread, Sandwiches, Or Pizza On The Ketogenic Diet

https://bit.ly/3h6rUGC

PROVEN-weight loss and body detoxifying supplements

https://bit.ly/2DQMkoA

Keto Resources

https://bit.ly/2CpPwqZ

Custom made keto Diet menus and shopping list just for you with the foods that you enjoy

https://bit.ly/2Cq4ehI

Do you have stored body fat that you have tried to get rid of in the past, but nothing worked?

https://bit.ly/3jiAfJ5

Over 40 Keto Solutions

https://bit.ly/398f8ol

Stuck in The Dreaded Keto Plateau? Take The Simple Keto Test.

https://bit.ly/2WBawSm

Ketogenic Accelerator

Gives you the benefits of a ketogenic diet without the strict carb restrictions

https://bit.ly/32E3MH8

Hot Skinny Tea - Detox Tea For Weight Loss!

https://bit.ly/2ZEfWh

Paleo Cookbook
470+ Recipes plus, A 10 Week Meal Plan And 2 Bonus ebooks!
https://bit.ly/39mqBAM

Keto Breads And Sweets
https://bit.ly/2Cn592z

100 healthy Raw Snacks And Sweets

Healthy, Natural, Sugar Free, No Cook Recipes
https://bit.ly/32CkXcd

Printed in Great Britain
by Amazon